The Yogurt Diet Cookbook

Harnessing the Power of Yogurt for a Healthy Lifestyle

Contents

Introduction to the Yogurt Diet Cookbook

In recent years, yogurt has gained immense popularity as a versatile and nutritious food. Not only is it delicious, but it also offers numerous health benefits. In this Yogurt Diet Cookbook, we will explore the many ways to incorporate yogurt into your daily meals, snacks, and desserts, while reaping the rewards of a balanced and healthy diet. Whether you're looking to shed a few pounds or simply maintain a nutritious lifestyle, this cookbook is your guide to making yogurt a central ingredient in your culinary adventures.

The Basics of Yogurt

Before diving into the recipes, it's essential to understand the different types of yogurt available. Greek yogurt, regular yogurt, low-fat, and non-fat variants all have unique characteristics. Greek yogurt, for example, is thicker and creamier due to the straining process that removes excess whey. Regular yogurt, on the other hand, is typically smoother and more liquid. Exploring these differences will help you choose the right yogurt for your specific needs and preferences.

Yogurt is not only delicious but also packed with nutrients. It is a good source of calcium, protein, and essential vitamins and minerals. It contains beneficial probiotics that support a healthy gut and digestion. Yogurt's versatility and nutritional value make it an ideal ingredient for a wide range of dishes.

Incorporating Yogurt into Your Daily Routine

Breakfast Ideas:

Start your day off right with yogurt-based breakfast options. Yogurt parfaits with fresh fruits and granola provide a delightful crunch and a burst of flavor. For a quick and refreshing breakfast, whip up a yogurt smoothie using various flavor combinations such as mixed berries, tropical fruits, or even a green smoothie packed with spinach and avocado. If you prefer a heartier breakfast, experiment with yogurt pancakes or waffles for a protein-rich twist on classic recipes.

Lunch and Dinner Recipes:

Yogurt can elevate your lunch and dinner dishes in many ways. Create creamy yogurt-based salad dressings using Greek yogurt, lemon juice, and herbs for a healthy alternative to store-bought dressings. Marinate grilled chicken or fish in a tangy yogurt mixture to tenderize and infuse flavors. Yogurt-based sauces and dips, such as tzatziki or raita, are perfect accompaniments for fresh vegetables or whole-grain crackers.

Snack Time: Yogurt makes for satisfying and nutritious snacks throughout the day. Prepare yogurt-based fruit popsicles by blending yogurt and your favorite fruits before freezing them in popsicle molds. Yogurt bowls with nuts and seeds offer a balanced snack packed with protein, healthy fats, and fiber. Additionally, whip up yogurt-based energy bites or bars for a quick and convenient snack to fuel your day.

Yogurt Desserts and Treats

While yogurt is often associated with breakfast and snacks, it can also be a star ingredient in desserts and treats.

Light and Healthy Desserts:

Indulge your sweet tooth guilt-free with yogurt-based desserts. Yogurt fruit tarts or pies offer a delightful combination of creamy yogurt and vibrant fruits atop a light crust. Frozen yogurt popsicles are a refreshing and low-calorie treat for hot summer days. For a light and fluffy dessert, experiment with yogurt-based mousse or pudding, flavored with cocoa, vanilla, or fruit puree.

Indulgent Treats with a Healthy Twist: If you're looking for a treat that satisfies your cravings while keeping health in mind, consider yogurt-based cheesecake or trifle.

These desserts replace heavy creams and sugars with yogurt, resulting in a lighter yet still indulgent taste. Yogurt ice cream recipes offer a healthier alternative to traditional ice creams, allowing you to enjoy creamy goodness with fewer calories and less added sugar. Yogurt-based smoothie bowls with toppings like fresh fruits, nuts, and granola create a decadent dessert-like experience that's as pleasing to the eyes as it is to the taste buds.

Introduction to the Yogurt Diet Cookbook

In recent years, yogurt has gained immense popularity as a versatile and nutritious food. Not only is it delicious, but it also offers numerous health benefits. In this Yogurt Diet Cookbook, we will explore the many ways to incorporate yogurt into your daily meals, snacks, and desserts, while reaping the rewards of a balanced and healthy diet. Whether you're looking to shed a few pounds or simply maintain a nutritious lifestyle, this cookbook is your guide to making yogurt a central ingredient in your culinary adventures.

The Basics of Yogurt

Before diving into the recipes, it's essential to understand the different types of yogurt available. Greek yogurt, regular yogurt, low-fat, and non-fat variants all have unique characteristics. Greek yogurt, for example, is thicker and creamier due to the straining process that removes excess whey. Regular yogurt, on the other hand, is typically smoother and more liquid. Exploring these differences will help you choose the right yogurt for your specific needs and preferences.

Yogurt is not only delicious but also packed with nutrients. It is a good source of calcium, protein, and essential vitamins and minerals. It contains beneficial probiotics that support a healthy gut and digestion. Yogurt's versatility and nutritional value make it an ideal ingredient for a wide range of dishes.

Incorporating Yogurt into Your Daily Routine

Breakfast Ideas: Start your day off right with yogurt-based breakfast options. Yogurt parfaits with fresh fruits and granola provide a delightful crunch and a burst of flavor. For a quick and refreshing breakfast, whip up a yogurt smoothie using various flavor combinations such as mixed berries, tropical fruits, or even a green smoothie packed with spinach and avocado. If you prefer a heartier breakfast, experiment with yogurt pancakes or waffles for a protein-rich twist on classic recipes.

Lunch and Dinner Recipes: Yogurt can elevate your lunch and dinner dishes in many ways. Create creamy yogurt-based salad dressings using Greek yogurt, lemon juice, and herbs for a healthy alternative to store-bought dressings. Marinate grilled chicken or fish in a tangy yogurt mixture to tenderize and infuse flavors. Yogurt-based sauces and dips, such as tzatziki or raita, are perfect accompaniments for fresh vegetables or whole-grain crackers.

Snack Time: Yogurt makes for satisfying and nutritious snacks throughout the day. Prepare yogurt-based fruit popsicles by blending yogurt and your favorite fruits before freezing them in popsicle molds. Yogurt bowls with nuts and seeds offer a balanced snack packed with protein, healthy fats, and fiber. Additionally, whip up yogurt-based energy bites or bars for a quick and convenient snack to fuel your day.

Yogurt Desserts and Treats

While yogurt is often associated with breakfast and snacks, it can also be a star ingredient in desserts and treats.

Light and Healthy Desserts: Indulge your sweet tooth guilt-free with yogurt-based desserts. Yogurt fruit tarts or pies offer a delightful combination of creamy yogurt and vibrant fruits atop a light crust. Frozen yogurt popsicles are a refreshing and low-calorie treat for hot summer days. For a light and fluffy dessert, experiment with yogurt-based mousse or pudding, flavored with cocoa, vanilla, or fruit puree.

Indulgent Treats with a Healthy Twist: If you're looking for a treat that satisfies your cravings while keeping health in mind, consider yogurt-based cheesecake or trifle. These desserts replace heavy creams and sugars with yogurt, resulting in a lighter yet still indulgent taste. Yogurt ice cream recipes offer a healthier alternative to traditional ice creams, allowing you to enjoy creamy goodness with fewer calories and less added sugar. Yogurt-based smoothie bowls with toppings like fresh fruits, nuts, and granola create a decadent dessert-like experience that's as pleasing to the eyes as it is to the taste buds.

Specialized Yogurt Diet Plans

For those looking to follow a yogurt-based diet plan, this cookbook offers specialized meal ideas to cater to specific goals.

One-Week Yogurt Diet Plan: Kickstart your yogurt diet journey with a comprehensive one-week meal plan. Each day features delicious and varied recipes that incorporate yogurt in different ways. From breakfast to dinner, the meal plans provide a balance of nutrients, ensuring you stay satisfied and nourished. The plan is accompanied by a shopping list and meal prep tips to make your journey seamless and enjoyable.

Yogurt Diet for Weight Loss:

Yogurt can be a valuable tool for weight loss due to its high protein content, which helps increase satiety. This section provides calorie-controlled meal ideas that center around yogurt as a central ingredient. These recipes are designed to keep you full and satisfied while supporting your weight loss goals. Additionally, strategies for portion control and mindful eating are included to promote a balanced and sustainable approach to weight management.

Yogurt Diet for Gut Health:

Yogurt's probiotic content makes it a fantastic choice for promoting a healthy gut microbiome. This section focuses on yogurt varieties that contain live and active cultures to support digestive health. Recipes featuring probiotic-rich ingredients such as fermented vegetables and kefir will help you nurture your gut and improve digestion.

To further enhance your yogurt journey, this cookbook provides additional resources such as tips for making homemade yogurt. By making your yogurt at home, you can control the quality and customize the flavors to suit your preferences. The section offers step-by-step instructions and valuable tips for successful yogurt-making adventures.

Conclusion

The Yogurt Diet Cookbook serves as your comprehensive guide to incorporating yogurt into your daily meals, snacks, and desserts. From breakfast to dinner, from weight loss to gut health, yogurt offers a myriad of possibilities to support your nutritional goals. With delicious and nutritious recipes, this cookbook empowers you to harness the power of yogurt for a healthy and fulfilling lifestyle. So, grab your spoon and join us on this exciting yogurt-filled journey towards a happier, healthier you.

1. Yogurt parfaits with fresh fruits and granola 2. Yogurt smoothies with various flavor combinations 3. Yogurt pancakes or waffles B. Lunch and Dinner Recipes 1. Creamy yogurt-based salad dressings 2. Yogurt-marinated grilled chicken or fish 3. Yogurt-based sauces and dips for vegetables or whole-grain crackers C. Snack Time 1. Yogurt-based fruit popsicles 2. Yogurt bowls

with nuts and seeds 3. Yogurt-based energy bites or bars IV. Yogurt Desserts and Treats A. Light and Healthy Desserts 1. Yogurt fruit tarts or pies 2. Frozen yogurt pops 3. Yogurt-based mousse or pudding B. Indulgent Treats with a Healthy Twist 1. Yogurt-based cheesecake or trifle 2. Yogurt ice cream recipes 3. Yogurt-based smoothie bowls with toppings

Breakfast Ideas

Yogurt Parfaits with Fresh Fruits and Granola Yogurt parfaits are a delightful and nutritious way to start your day. Layer creamy yogurt with a variety of fresh fruits such as berries, sliced bananas, or diced mangoes. Add a crunchy element by sprinkling granola or toasted nuts between the layers. The combination of creamy yogurt, juicy fruits, and crunchy toppings creates a balanced and satisfying breakfast that will keep you energized throughout the morning.

Yogurt Smoothies with Various Flavor Combinations Yogurt smoothies are a refreshing and versatile option for breakfast. Blend together your favorite fruits, such as strawberries, blueberries, or peaches, with yogurt and a liquid of your choice, such as milk or almond milk. You can also add a handful of spinach or kale for an extra boost of nutrients. Experiment with different flavor combinations by adding a touch of honey, a sprinkle of cinnamon, or a spoonful of nut butter. The result is a creamy and nutritious smoothie that will kickstart your day on a delicious note.

Yogurt Pancakes or Waffles If you're in the mood for a more indulgent breakfast, yogurt pancakes or waffles are a fantastic option. Simply add yogurt to your favorite pancake or waffle batter recipe to create a moist and fluffy texture. The yogurt adds a tangy flavor while keeping the pancakes or waffles light and airy. Serve them with fresh fruits, a drizzle of honey or maple syrup, and a dollop of yogurt for a delightful breakfast treat that the whole family will love.

Lunch and Dinner Recipes

Creamy Yogurt-Based Salad Dressings Enhance your salads with creamy yogurt-based dressings. Combine Greek yogurt with fresh herbs, lemon juice, garlic, and a touch of olive oil for a tangy and flavorful dressing. You can also experiment with different herbs and spices like dill, cilantro, or paprika to create unique variations. Pour the dressing over a bed of mixed greens, vegetables, and protein such as grilled chicken or chickpeas for a satisfying and healthy lunch or dinner option.

Yogurt-Marinated Grilled Chicken or Fish Elevate the flavor and juiciness of your grilled chicken or fish by marinating them in yogurt. Mix yogurt with spices like paprika, cumin, turmeric, and a squeeze of lemon juice to create a flavorful marinade. Coat the chicken or fish in the yogurt mixture and let it marinate for a few hours or overnight. When you're ready to cook, grill the marinated protein until it's tender and juicy.

The yogurt marinade adds a tangy and moist element to the dish, making it a mouthwatering and healthy choice for lunch or dinner.

Yogurt-Based Sauces and Dips for Vegetables or Whole-Grain Crackers Yogurt-based sauces and dips are versatile accompaniments that can elevate your lunch or dinner options. Create a refreshing tzatziki sauce by combining Greek yogurt, cucumber, garlic, lemon juice, and dill. It pairs perfectly with grilled vegetables, falafel, or whole-grain crackers. You can also create a creamy yogurt-based dip by mixing yogurt with roasted red peppers, garlic, and a touch of olive oil. This dip is ideal for snacking with fresh vegetables or spreading on whole-grain bread.

Snack Time

Yogurt-Based Fruit Popsicles During the warmer months, indulge in yogurt-based fruit popsicles for a healthy and cooling snack. Blend together yogurt and your favorite fruits, such as strawberries, mangoes, or kiwis. Pour the mixture into popsicle molds and insert sticks. Freeze them until solid, and you'll have a delicious and guilt-free treat that's bursting with fruity flavors.

Yogurt Bowls with Nuts and Seeds For a quick and satisfying snack, create yogurt bowls with nuts and seeds. Start with a base of creamy yogurt and top it with a variety of nuts, such as almonds, walnuts, or pistachios, for added crunch and healthy fats. Sprinkle chia seeds, flaxseeds, or pumpkin seeds for an extra nutritional boost. Drizzle a small amount of honey or maple syrup for sweetness, and you have a nourishing and filling snack that will keep you energized throughout the day.

Yogurt-Based Energy Bites or Bars Prepare homemade yogurt-based energy bites or bars for a convenient on-the-go snack. Combine yogurt with oats, nut butter, honey, and a mix of nuts, seeds, and dried fruits. Form the mixture into bite-sized balls or press it into a baking dish to create bars. Refrigerate or freeze until firm, and you'll have a nutritious snack packed with protein, fiber, and natural sweetness.

Incorporating yogurt into your breakfast, lunch, dinner, and snack time will not only add a creamy and tangy element to your meals but also provide you with essential nutrients. With these versatile and delicious yogurt-based recipes, you can enjoy a balanced and wholesome diet while savoring the benefits of yogurt's rich flavor and healthful properties.

Yogurt 101: Nutrition Facts and Health Benefits

Yogurt is one of the most popular fermented dairy products in the world, made by adding live bacteria to milk.

It has been eaten for thousands of years and is frequently used as part of a meal or snack, as well as a component of sauces and desserts.

In addition, yogurt contains beneficial bacteria and may function as a probiotic, providing a variety of health benefits above and beyond plain milk.

Most yogurt is white and thick, but many commercial brands are artificially colored.

This article tells you everything you need to know about yogurt.

Nutrition Facts

The nutrients in 3.5 ounces (100 grams) of plain, whole-milk yogurt are detailed below.

Nutrition Facts: Yogurt, plain, whole milk — 100 grams

Nutrient Amount

Calories 61

Water 88%

Protein 3.5 g

Carbs 4.7 g

Sugar 4.7 g

Fiber 0 g

Fat 3.3 g

Protein

Yogurt is a rich source of protein.

One cup (245 grams) of plain yogurt made from whole milk packs about 8.5 grams of protein.

The protein content of commercial yogurt is sometimes higher than in milk because dry milk may be added to yogurt during processing.

Protein in yogurt is either whey or casein, depending on its solubility in water.

Water-soluble milk proteins are called whey proteins, whereas insoluble milk proteins are called caseins.

Both casein and whey are nutritionally excellent, rich in essential amino acids, and easy to digest.

Casein

Most of the proteins in yogurt (80%) are caseins. Alpha-casein is the most abundant.

Casein increases your absorption of minerals like calcium and phosphorus and promotes lower blood pressure.

Whey

Whey accounts for 20% of the protein in yogurt.

It is very high in branched-chain amino acids (BCAAs), such as valine, leucine, and isoleucine.

Whey protein has long been popular amongst bodybuilders and athletes.

In addition, consumption of whey protein supplements may provide various health benefits, promoting weight loss and lower blood pressure.

Fat

The amount of fat in yogurt depends on the type of milk it's made from.

Yogurt can be produced from all kinds of milk — whole, low-fat, or fat-free. Most yogurt sold in the United States is either low-fat or fat-free.

The fat content can range from 0.4% in nonfat yogurt to 3.3% or more in full-fat yogurt.

Most of the fat in yogurt is saturated (70%), but it also contains a fair amount of monounsaturated fat.

Milk fat is unique because it provides as many as 400 different types of fatty acids.

Ruminant Trans Fats in Yogurt

Yogurt hosts trans fats called ruminant trans fats or dairy trans fats.

Unlike trans fats found in some processed food products, ruminant trans fats are considered beneficial.

The most abundant ruminant trans fats in yogurt are vaccenic acid and conjugated linoleic acid (CLA). Yogurt may have even more CLA than milk.

Researchers believe that CLA has various health benefits — but taking large doses of CLA supplements may have harmful metabolic consequences .

Carbs

Carbs in plain yogurt occur mainly as simple sugars called lactose (milk sugar) and galactose.

However, the lactose content of yogurt is lower than in milk. This is because bacterial fermentation results in lactose breakdown.

When lactose is broken down, it forms galactose and glucose. The glucose is mostly converted to lactic acid, the substance that contributes the sour flavor to yogurt and other fermented milk products.

Most yogurts also contain considerable amounts of added sweeteners — usually sucrose (white sugar) — alongside various flavorings.

As a result, the amount of sugar in yogurt is highly variable and may range from 4.7% to 18.6% or higher.

SUMMARY

Yogurt is a great source of high-quality protein, offers various amounts of fat, and contains small amounts of lactose. Many brands are also high in added sugar and flavorings.

Vitamins and Minerals

Full-fat yogurt contains almost every single nutrient you need.

However, nutritional value varies substantially among different types of yogurt.

For example, the nutritional value may depend on the types of bacteria used in the fermentation process.

The following vitamins and minerals are found in particularly high amounts in conventional yogurt made from whole milk:

• Vitamin B12. This nutrient is found almost exclusively in animal foods.

• Calcium. Milk products are excellent sources of easily absorbable calcium.

• Phosphorus. Yogurt is a good source of phosphorus, an essential mineral that plays an important role in biological processes.

• Riboflavin. Milk products are the main source of riboflavin (vitamin B2) in the modern diet.

SUMMARY

Yogurt is an excellent source of several vitamins and minerals, such as vitamin B12, calcium, phosphorus, and riboflavin.

Probiotics

Probiotics are live bacteria that have beneficial health effects.

These friendly bacteria are found in fermented milk products, such as yogurt with live and active cultures.

The main probiotics in fermented milk products are lactic acid bacteria and bifidobacteria.

Probiotics have many beneficial health effects, depending on the species and the amount taken.

- Enhanced immune system. Studies indicate that probiotic bacteria may promote enhanced immunity.

- Lower cholesterol. Regular intake of certain types of probiotics and fermented milk products may lower blood cholestero).

- Vitamin synthesis. Bifidobacteria can synthesize or make available many kinds of vitamins, including thiamine, niacin, folate, and vitamins B6, B12, and K (22).

- Digestive health. Fermented milk containing bifidobacterium may promote digestive well-being and relieve the symptoms of irritable bowel syndrome (IBS).

- Protection against diarrhea. Probiotics may help treat diarrhea caused by antibiotics.

- Protection against constipation. Several studies suggest that regular consumption of yogurt fermented with bifidobacterium may reduce constipation.

- Improved lactose digestibility. Probiotic bacteria have been shown to improve the digestion of lactose, lessening the symptoms of lactose intolerance.

These health benefits do not always apply to yogurt because some types of yogurt have been pasteurized after the probiotic bacteria were added — thus neutralizing the bacteria.

For this reason, it is best to choose yogurt with active and live cultures.

SUMMARY

Yogurts with live and active cultures contain probiotic bacteria that may improve digestive health.

Health Benefits of Yogurt

The health effects of milk and fermented dairy products like yogurt have been widely studied.

Probiotic yogurt can provide numerous impressive health benefits that go well beyond that of non-fermented milk.

Digestive Health

Probiotic yogurt is associated with a variety of digestive health benefits.

Regular consumption of yogurt with live and active cultures may help treat antibiotic-associated diarrhea by restoring balance in your intestinal flora.

In addition, probiotic yogurt with bifidobacteria may lessen the symptoms of IBS and help reduce constipation.

Probiotics may also alleviate the symptoms of lactose intolerance by improving your digestion of lactose.

Osteoporosis and Bone Health

Osteoporosis is a condition characterized by weak and brittle bones.

It is common among older adults and is the main risk factor for bone fractures in this age group.

Dairy products have long been considered protective against osteoporosis.

In fact, dairy is associated with higher bone density, an effect linked to its high calcium and protein content.

Blood Pressure

Abnormally high blood pressure is one of the main risk factors for heart disease.

Studies suggest that regular consumption of yogurt may lower blood pressure in people who already have high readings.

However, this effect is not limited to yogurt. Studies on intake of other milk products have provided similar results.

SUMMARY

Consumption of probiotic yogurt may improve gut health, reduce your risk of osteoporosis, and combat high blood pressure.

Potential Downsides

Yogurt may cause adverse effects in certain people — especially in anyone who's lactose intolerant or allergic to milk proteins.

Lactose Intolerance

Yogurt contains less milk sugar (lactose) than milk.

That's because some of the lactose in milk breaks down into glucose and galactose during yogurt production.

Therefore, it is better tolerated by people with lactose intolerance.

However, probiotic bacteria may also help by improving your ability to digest lactose.

Notably, lactose-intolerant individuals tolerate yogurt with added lactose better than milk with the same amount of lactose.

Milk Allergy

Milk allergy is rare and more common among children than adults. It is triggered by the milk proteins — whey and casein — found in all milk products.

Therefore, yogurt should be avoided by people who have a milk allergy.

Added Sugar

Keep in mind that many low-fat yogurts have copious amounts of added sugar.

High sugar intake linked to numerous health problems, such as type 2 diabetes and heart.

For this reason, it's best to read the label and avoid yogurt that has sugar — usually in the form of sucrose or high-fructose corn syrup — in its ingredients.

SUMMARY

Yogurt may pose health risks for anyone with lactose intolerance or a milk allergy.

What's more, commercial varieties often include significant amounts of added sugar, which can be harmful when consumed in excess.

The Bottom Line

Yogurt is a dairy product made by fermenting milk.

Natural probiotic yogurt with live and active cultures is one of the healthiest dairy products, especially when it's free of added sugar.

It has various digestive benefits and may reduce blood pressure and your risk of osteoporosis.

www.ingramcontent.com/pod-product-compliance
Lightning Source LLC
Chambersburg PA
CBHW061935270726
48660CB00007BA/2729